Failure-Free Activities for the Alzheimer's Patient

A Guidebook for Caregivers

Carmel Sheridan, M.A.

Cottage Books
Oakland,
California.

Copyright   © 1987   by Cottage Books

Library of Congress Cataloging in Publication Data

Main entry under title:

Failure - Free Activities for the Alzheimer's Patient
    Sheridan, Carmel B.

1. Alzheimer's disease. 2. Activities 3. Home care services.
4. Aged—Home care. 5. Nursing home care.   I. Title
LCCN 87-70051
ISBN 0-943873-05-3

Printed in the United States of America

This book is dedicated to caregivers everywhere who shoulder the burden of Alzheimer's disease.

Note to Readers

Alzheimer's disease affects both men and women and to simplify reading, the masculine pronouns *he* and *his* and the feminine pronouns *she* and *hers* are used in alternate chapters.

The purpose of this book is to describe activities which can bring moment-to-moment satisfaction to the Alzheimer's patient. <u>Not all</u> suggestions will be appropriate for all patients. It is the responsibility of each reader to exercise good judgement in using the activities herein. The book is not intended to provide medical advice. The services of a competent professional should be obtained when medical or other specific advice is needed. No responsibility can be assumed by the publishers for any loss or damage alleged to be caused directly or indirectly by the information contained in this book.

Table of Contents

Acknowledgements

My thanks to the staff, volunteers and participants of the Alzheimer's day-care program at St. Joseph's Center in Oakland, especially to the director, Rita Sklar.

To the Alzheimer's Disease and Related Disorders Association (ADRDA) for information and assistance given over the years.

To the staff members of the Psychology Department, University College, Galway, Ireland.

I would like to express my warmest thanks to Rachel Laurgaard in Oakland for all her encouragement and enthusiasm for this book.

My thanks go to Dr. Eleanor Levine and Robert Heaney for giving me a quiet, uninterrupted work-space and much encouragement.

To Suzanne Cronin for her concise reading of the manuscript, and her helpful editorial comments.

My deepest thanks go to Eddie for his unflagging support and for the perceptive and creative way he helped shape the material.

A special ' thank you' to my family and friends for their support.

Introduction

For the person affected by Alzheimer's disease, the day is often filled with failures, mistakes and obstacles. These occur as a result of a reduced capacity in many areas, brought about by changes in the brain. During the early stages of the disease especially, the inability to remember and communicate things is a terrible source of frustration and stress. Without adequate memory and a capacity to know and interpret everyday happenings, the world for the victim becomes a frightening and threatening place to be. As the disease advances, the opportunity for success and a feeling of self-worth is further limited. Failure becomes an all-too-familiar experience; even in little things, the Alzheimer's patient fails repeatedly. And every caregiver knows the frustration and helplessness that ensue.

The aim of this book is to offer simple activities which help reinforce the patient's self-esteem while relieving boredom and frustration at the same time. This, for the caregiver, involves being alert to the preserved abilities of the patient, and helping her develop and use the skills she still has. The more involved Alzheimer's patients remain with the world around them, the more resourceful they become at finding ways to keep that world from slipping away.

The activities described here may be used by all who come in contact with the Alzheimer's patient: the family caregiver, the companion, the nurse's aide or the occasional visitor. They are described as **failure-free activities** because they are adapted to suit the needs and capacities of the person with memory loss, and are to be used in a way that will enable the person to succeed.

Used appropriately, activities provide moment-to-moment satisfaction and raise self-esteem. They help nurture the person by removing the focus from the **disability** onto preserved abilities. By allowing the patient to have a meaningful role, be it washing the dishes, dusting, or singing along to old tunes on the radio, the patient's self-confidence is built up.

Caregivers can help slow the consequences of the disease by allowing the patient perform at her fullest potential. This involves recognizing whatever skills and interests are retained and helping the patient to capitalize on these. The emphasis is on assets rather than deficits, and the patient is helped to use the abilities which remain. Chores and simple activities can be sensitively set at a level which does not place the person in a position of failure.

Which activities work best?

Only time and experience will show which of the activities described in this book are the most suitable for your relative. Since there is very little evidence to suggest which activities work best, a trial-and-error approach, with adjustments based on observations, is essential.

The findings of one survey, however, may be worth keeping in mind as you set about planning activities at home. **Nancy Mace** surveyed 346 day-care centers nationwide and reported that the most successful activities with victims of memory loss were those which:

- Take advantage of old skills

- Offer social interaction
  (sing-alongs, pets, visits from children.)

- Allow considerable physical activity
  (physical exercise, active games, walks and outings)

- Support cognitive functions
  (reality orientation, reminiscence, and listening to music)

In the survey, the following specific activities were identified as being most successful (those which participants seemed to enjoy most):

Sing-alongs	Active games
Physical exercise	Outings
Walks	Listening to music
Reminiscence	Reality orientation
Visits from children	Visits from pets

The centers surveyed reported that the above activities were more successful than quiet games (e.g. bingo), and activities that require fine motor and language skills (e.g. crafts and current events discussions).

Features of Activities

The choice of activities is extremely important. Most A.D. patients are aware of their memory loss and failing in a simple activity will only add to their frustration. The following guidelines then should help family members in their use of the activities described in this book:

Simplicity The activities in this book are short, simple and have few verbal instructions.When using them bear in mind that their simplicity is the key to their success. Keep them simple !

Duration Because the person with A.D. has a reduced attention span, the optimum time for any activity is from twenty to thirty minutes.

Distraction   If the patient becomes frustrated or upset, discontinue or switch to another activity.

Flexibility   Be creative and flexible in your approach. If one activity doesn't work, try another tactic.

Level of Activities   Keep activities on an adult level for as long as possible, but bear in mind that as the disease progresses, childrens' picture books and games may be useful.

Music

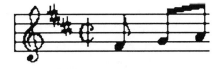

Music

The most successful activity for the Alzheimer's patient is usually one which incorporates music. Families often comment that long after the meaning of other social cues have been forgotten, their relative still enjoys old familiar songs and melodies. In fact, the centers surveyed by **Nancy Mace** rated sing-alongs as the most popular activity with victims of memory loss.

Unlike most other activities, music doesn't require a long attention span or good coordination. Since no risky materials are involved (as is the case, for example, with arts and crafts) music is also a relatively safe activity. Equally important, music is by its very nature failure-free and undemanding.

Music can be a valuable resource in recalling past pleasures. A wealth of associations, imagery, thoughts, and feelings may be sparked off by a single song. Old songs and melodies are especially useful for eliciting memories and triggering the feelings that accompanied them. The familiar strains of "Silent Night" or "School Days" are simple examples of how music can be used as an access to past experiences and events. The Alzheimer's patient will think of Christmas when she hears "Silent Night." Likewise, she will associate childhood or adolescence with the piece entitled "School Days."

As well as eliciting memories, music can also stir up new thoughts and feelings. Most of the time, we listen to music for a reason: to cheer up, slow down, to relax, or to feel in harmony with those around us. Music can have the same benefit for the Alzheimer's patient; moods can be created or changed. Different types of music can touch parts of the self which may be unreachable by any other means.

Making Music

Many patients may still be able to play a musical instrument if they learned the skill earlier in life. This is because lifelong hobbies and pastimes which were always a source of enjoyment are retained the longest, even in very impaired patients. Families have told of relatives who retained the ability to play the piano well into the moderate stages of the disease.

If your relative retains such an ability, provide ample opportunity for her to enjoy it for as long as possible. Some families recommend using music-makers such as small portable electric keyboards, which allow the patient to create pleasing sounds. They also have the added advantage of letting the caregiver know where the patient is by the sounds.

Portable Keyboard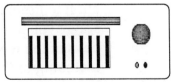

Listening to Music

Listening to music can help a person with A.D. to reach thoughts and feelings more easily. Once you have identified the patient's preferred music tastes, you can supply appropriate background music. Tastes may vary from folk, popular, jazz, country and western, and classical to religious music. A portable "walkman" radio or cassette player with earphones may work well. Keep the music low, and try to ensure it's in keeping with the patient's preferences (no heavy rock!). Play music that evokes pleasant associations, memories, thoughts and images. If the patient is bilingual, music and songs from her native culture will be enjoyable.

Sing-Alongs

Sing-alongs can be very enjoyable for the A.D. patient and two or three people can generate enough energy for a successful sing-along. Encourage the patient to hum or sing a favorite tune. Acknowledge her presence by singing her favorite song. Nearly everyone has one, even if they don't realize it! Singing a person's favorite song and dedicating it to them is a special way of saying "We're glad you're here."

Use songs which will help to promote orientation to time, place and person. Think of all the songs you know which refer to the weather, the days of the week, the months of the year. Listening to these songs at relevant times may help keep the patient oriented.

- Select songs with place names to facilitate orientation to place.

Chicago, Chicago	Deep in the Heart of Texas
Tennessee Waltz	North to Alaska
Yellow Rose of Texas	Black Hills of Dakota
South of the Border	Off to Alabama
Moonlight in Vermont	The Old Cotton Fields Back Home
Red River Valley	I Left my Heart in San Francisco

- Select songs with personal names—this will help to acknowledge the patient's presence. Here are some ideas:

If You Knew Susie	Danny Boy
Rambling Rose	Joe Hill
Ramona	Billy Boy
Peggy O'Neill	Alexander's Ragtime Band
Oh Marie	John Brown's Body
Charmaine	Jacob's Ladder
Irene Goodnight	Casey Jones
Daisy, Daisy	

- Here are a few suggestions for seasonal songs:

Springtime in the Rockies	Those Autumn Leaves
Lazy Days of Summer	April in Paris
April Showers	White Christmas

Rhythm Instruments

Rhythm instruments can be used to accompany singing sessions. Simple instruments can be made from ordinary, easy-to-find, inexpensive things. Drums can be made from various containers including cereal boxes, coffee cans, or potato chip cans. They don't have to be round.

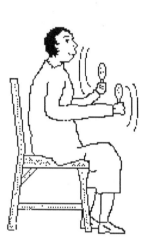 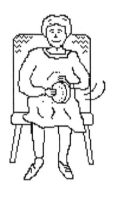 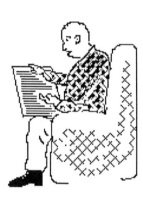

Shaking dry beans or uncooked rice in a can will produce an interesting sound, as will rattling aluminum foil, or knocking wooden dowels together.

Movement to Music

Dancing or moving to music will give everyone a chance to touch, to hold hands and get close. The patient may dance spontaneously to music, or with prompting may move to music with a strong beat—such as military marches and country dance tunes.

Even those who are not ambulant will find therapy in having a caregiver maneuver their chairs around in rhythm to the music. Simple, gentle movements can be carried out even with the person seated. Following are examples of songs which are particularly suited to move to. Use appropriate motions for particular songs.

If You're Happy and You Know it..

Hokey Pokey

Shoe the Donkey

Blowing Bubbles

Michael Row the Boat Ashore

When the Saints Come Marching In

He's Got the Whole World in His Hands

Do the Locomotion

Row, Row, Row Your Boat

Exercise

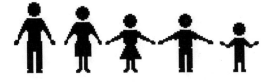

Exercise

Overall activity is often reduced in Alzheimer's disease so that even those who were once fit and active are reduced to leading sedentary lives. Eventually, people affected may become reluctant to move at all; others may pace restlessly.

Some form of exercise should be encouraged early on in the disease to improve the patient's muscle tone and maintain range of motion. Exercise also helps confused people to sleep better at night. Perhaps of most importance to the caregiver is the fact that adequate exercise helps relieve feelings of tension and anxiety and patients are sometimes much calmer as a result. Some researchers have in fact shown that exercise as brief as a fifteen-minute walk has the same effect as a tranquilizer on muscular tension. Exercise then can have both physical and psychological benefits, as indicated below:

Benefits of Exercise

- Regular exercise helps promote general fitness and mobility.

- Exercise reduces tension and provides a physical outlet for the discharge of energy.

- Body self-awareness can be enhanced through exercise.

- The patient can get pleasure and satisfaction from movement and can work through anger by physical means.

- Exercise in a group situation with family or friends can facilitate interaction and build group cohesion.

Walking

If ever a fitness activity were taken for granted, it is the daily stroll! It's safe and usually non-threatening, and you can step right outside your front door and begin. Walking is in fact the primary exercise for 55 million Americans, according to a National Parks Services survey.

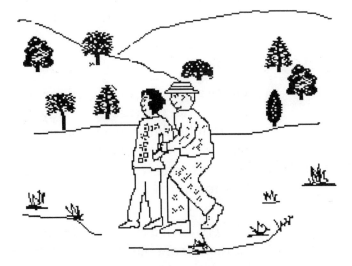

Try getting into the habit of going for a daily walk with the patient. Select a peaceful route; perhaps a boardwalk, beach or quiet park. It will be easier for the confused person if you go at the same time each day, use the same door and take the same route. Make sure both of you wear low-heeled comfortable shoes with an arched support. Since the patient may not be able to seek out experiences to stimulate his senses, it will help if you point out what he may not be able to notice by himself: something pretty to see, to hear, to taste, to smell or to touch. Notice the sensations he seems to enjoy so you can draw attention to them again and again.

Walking can be an everyday activity, come rain, hail or shine. When the weather is poor, walking briskly indoors to the beat of music can be fun, and good exercise too! Or you can drive to a shopping complex and window shop.

Active Games

Physical games, simplified for the benefit of the patient, can provide a fun way to exercise for all the family. This can also be a good time for family members and the confused person to share closeness and affection without having to talk too much.

Bat the Balloon
Players form a circle and the balloon is batted at random from one person to the next. It is kept circulating for as long as the energy lasts. This game can be varied and adapted to suit the ability of the patient.

Pass the Ball Players sit or stand around in a circle at arm's length from each other. The leader hands the ball to any one player and asks him to pass it to a person on either side. While passing it, he says the person's name. The ball is passed around from person to person for two to three rounds.

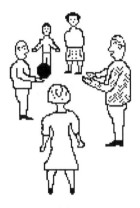

Catch the Bag This is a simplified version of the usual "Catch," suitable for two players. Instead of using a ball, a small bean bag is hung from the ceiling and swings back and forth betwen two players. This is an enjoyable activity for young people to share with the patient and it can be played while seated.

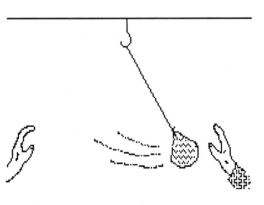

23

Bowling   Bowling is a wonderful failure-free game which can be played by arranging plastic skittles or ten pin bowls on the floor. The ball is rolled to the patient who aims for the pins. This is a useful game for exercising the arms and trunk since the player must bend to catch the ball and flex the muscles to roll it to the pins.

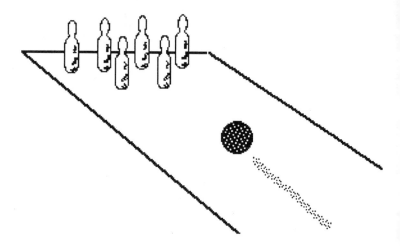

Bowling can also be played by arranging skittles on a long table of suitable height. A trap for the ball can be made at the end of the table. If the patient is wheelchair-bound, a simple cardboard guide can be made to rest on her knees so that she can roll the ball down the guide towards the pins.

Shuffle-board
In this game, small wooden discs are pushed with a shuffleboard stick as far as they can go on the shuffleboard base. At the Oakland Day Care Center, this was one of the most popular games and was often played outdoors on sunny summer afternoons. The entire kit, including the sticks and wooden discs may be made quite easily. The base can be made from heavy oil cloth or plastic and marked into segments.

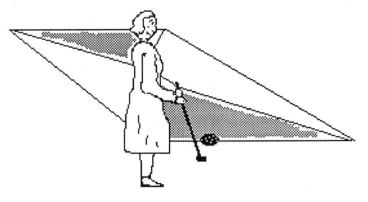

Basketball
A simplified version of basketball can be played where the patient tosses a rubber ball into a laundry basket. The caregiver retrieves the ball after each pitch and rolls it back to the patient.

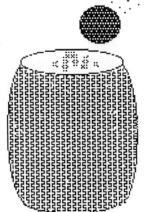

Circle Toss Three concentric circles are marked on a board, large piece of plastic or cardboard, which is placed on the floor. The patient sits or stands outside the outer circle and tosses three bean-bags at the bull's-eye which is the inner circle.

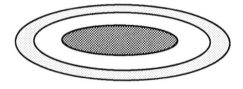

Beanbag Toss Prop a heavy board with large holes against the wall. Ask the patient to pitch a beanbag into the holes. This activity can be done from a sitting or standing position.

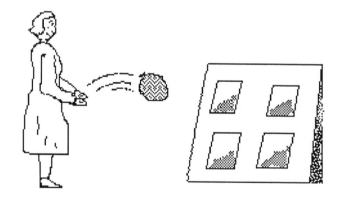

Domestic Exercises

Taking part in household chores can give the patient a chance to exercise and a sense of doing something useful. Ideally, you may be able to establish a routine of household activities based on what was enjoyable in the past. Select chores which are relatively simple, repetitive and hazard-free. For example, at mealtimes perhaps the patient could contribute by:

- Handing out paper napkins
- Putting out the placemats
- Sorting and putting away cutlery after meal

Repetitive actions are a common characteristic of A.D. behavior. You can capitalize on this pattern by selecting household activities which involve repetitive movements. These should be simple enough to be completed by the patient. Remember it isn't so important that the job be done perfectly—but it should give a sense of accomplishment to the patient.
Here are some ideas:

- Raking leaves
- Dusting
- Vacuum cleaning
- Mowing the lawn
- Mopping the floor
- Whipping cream
- Beating eggs
- Picking up fallen fruit

Light Body Exercise

Confused people often enjoy doing light body exercises as part of a group or with a partner. When you try these exercises, teach each one by demonstration and have the patient imitate what you do, gently guiding him if necessary. If he has arthritis or any other medical condition that makes movement a problem, ask a physical therapist to recommend special exercises for him.

To minimize confusion, try to exercise at the same time each day for about ten minutes and follow the same sequence of activities. Start from the head and work all the way down to the feet, beginning with a gradual warm-up to loosen tight muscles. Light rhythmic clapping and stamping are good warm-up exercises. Then continue:

Head
- Look straight ahead

- Bend ear to shoulder and hold

- Repeat for other side of body

Face
- Give a broad smile— show your teeth
- Raise your eyebrows
- Pucker your lips— kiss
- Blow out a mouthful of air

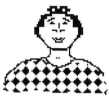

Shoulders
- Hold arms at side
- Raise shoulders up to earlobes— shrug
- Relax shoulders

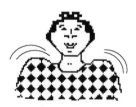

Arms
- Stretch both arms straight in front. Hold palms up.
- Move arms upward as far as possible
- Lower arms slowly to lap

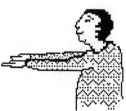

Hand Exercises

Hand and arm exercise can be got through rolling playdough and tying simple knots. Both activities should always be supervised.

Playdough
- Show the patient how to shape playdough into a long roll.

- Then roll it back and forth, from palm to fingertips

- Fold it in double and repeat the preceeding

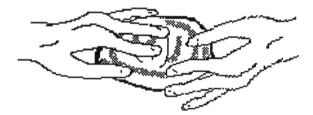

Tying
- Tie and untie simple knots in soft cord and steps.

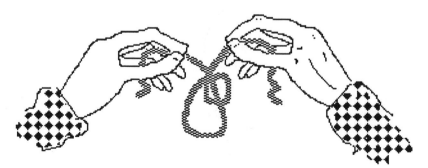

Chair Exercises

The following are a few simple exercises which can be done from a sitting position. Begin slowly, asking the patient to imitate you.

Upper Body

- Sit upright and spread knees

- Slowly bend forward from the waist

- Reach hands toward floor and hold for a count of two

- Slowly return to straight position

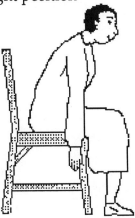

Legs

- Place feet flat on floor

- Raise one leg in front as far as you can

- Hold for a count of two

- Return foot to floor and relax

Knees

- Place feet flat on floor, and arms by side

- Bend knee and raise foot slightly from floor

- Return foot to floor

- Repeat with other leg

Feet

- Place feet flat on floor

- Lift one foot off the floor, then the other Stamp gently in marching fashion

- Place both feet on floor again and relax

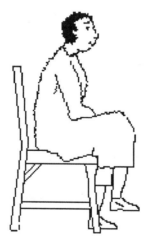

Conclude exercise session with a slow stretch to cool down:

- Sit straight with arms on lap

- Slowly raise arms above head and take a deep breath

- Slowly lower arms and exhale

- Relax

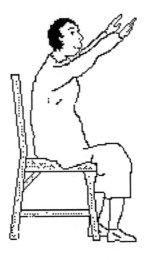

Exercise to Music

It is often helpful to exercise to music and use props such as balls, wooden dowels or elastic ropes. Both music and exercise involve rhythm, tempo and movement. The rhythm and tempo of a piece of music may help cue the timing and pacing of movements such as leg lifts or stretches. Swaying to music, clapping hands, or tapping feet are all simple exercises which stimulate the flow of oxygen to the brain.

Use soft background music which will not interfere with the patient's ability to hear and process your instructions. Have him imitate what you do and if he gets stuck or has trouble, try helping him move gently.

Making Exercise Failure - Free

- Begin with simple, easy-to-follow exercises and limit the length of time spent at each to five minutes.

- Move into each new exercise slowly. Monitor the patient's progress and stop if he seems to tire or lose interest.

- Simplify instructions— don't give directions which distinguish between the right and left sides of the body.

- Avoid using exercises which require the patient to hold his breath too long or stamp his feet energetically as these will cause strain or overexertion

- Stop and rest after every five minutes or so and have a chat. Talking and having fun will make an activity more enjoyable and double the benefit.

- Watch for signs of overexertion. Suggest that the patient slow down if he seems to be overdoing it.

Food Preparation

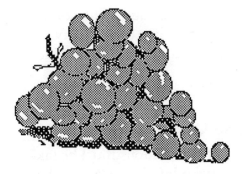

Food Preparation

Many Alzheimer patients are able to do simple food preparation, and all are adept at sampling the finished dish! At the Oakland Day Care Center, cooking and food preparation was found to be a very popular activity. Women generally respond especially well to this activity, probably because food preparation has been a large part of their active lives. Memory of this involvement is stimulated through sight, sound, smell and taste. At the same time, this activity emphasizes sequence, counting and object identification.

Making Sessions Failure-Free

Certain precautions must be taken to make this activity both failure-free and hazard-free.

- Each task must be broken up into its smallest components and continuous direction given on each step. For example:
  "Break the eggs—now beat them."
  "Wash the vegetable—now slice it."

- The exercise should also be quick to complete because of the patient's short attention span.

- As few ingredients as possible should be set out at any one time, and the patient should be familiar with those used.

- Examine activities for potential hazards before beginning. Sharp instruments should be put out of reach.

- If an activity calls for canned ingredients, cans should be opened by the caregiver.The contents should be put into a bowl and the container trashed.

- On no account should the patient be allowed to use a stove or barbeque.

Activity Ideas

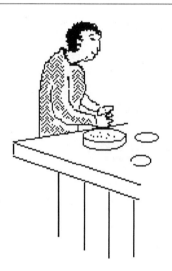

Cookie Baking With some supervision, cookie baking is an activity well within the grasp of many patients. Using a favorite crispy cookie recipe, jobs can be assigned on the basis of the patient's ability. Specifically, ingredients must be measured, sifted, beaten together, and the batter put on trays.

Those are the basic steps involved, and the patient may be able to do only one or all of them. The other steps involved, such as putting cookies into the oven, have an element of risk, and should be done only by the caregiver.

Salads With your assistance, the patient may be able to help prepare a full salad such as cold meat, vegetable, fruit, tuna or salmon. Whatever type of salad is being prepared, the same basic steps are involved. The patient might assist in washing the lettuce and other vegetables, and tossing the salad with dressing.

Cakes Cake decoration can bring almost immediate gratification because of instant colorful results. The patient may be able to help mix the icing, color and flavor it, and put the decorations on top of a ready-baked cake. Cakes can also be baked quite easily using cake mixes which just need water, milk or eggs.

Desserts Various desserts can be made using assorted canned or fresh fruit and served with whipped cream or yogurt. Pastry shells filled with fruit and covered with topping make an appetizing dish. Desserts which only need cold milk can be served up with jelly.

Snacks Sandwiches with cheese spreads can be made quite easily. Vegetable dips are easily prepared and look appetizing and colorful. Crackers and cheese and other such snacks need minimal preparation.

Simple Recipes

You will find simple recipes in cookbooks, magazines and newspapers which can be adapted to involve the patient in some or all of the steps in preparation. Again, the level of involvement will depend on the patient's capabilities. Supervision is very important and stove top and oven procedures should only be carried out by the caregiver.

The following recipes are quick and easy to prepare. You can compile a program of simple recipes of your own.

Kedegree This is an interesting recipe which tastes delightful and can be made quite easily. You will need the following ingredients and the rice and eggs should be prepared in advance and allowed to cool. The fish should be drained and left on a plate. The patient will be able to wash the vegetables and maybe prepare them under supervision. To prepare the dish you will need a large bowl and wooden spoon.

3 cups of cooked rice.
1 can of salmon or tuna, drained
1 half cup of chopped green pepper
1 half cup of chopped red pepper
3 green onions chopped
1 tomato cut in wedges
2 hard boiled eggs
1 half cup of mayonnaise
seasoning to taste

The ingredients are mixed together in a large bowl in the sequence listed above—first the rice, then fish, peppers and so on.When the kedegree is thoroughly mixed, it is chilled for an hour or so. Served on a bed of lettuce and garnished with chives and lemon wedges, this dish also gives the patient good involvement in the presentation and serving activities.

Nutritious Peanut Butter Snack

You will need the ingredients below and a large bowl and wooden spoon for this recipe.

I cup of peanut butter
I tbs. of margarine
1 cup of nonfat dry milk
1 half cup of chopped nuts
1 half cup of raisins
1 half cup of dates
2 cups of cracker crumbs

The caregiver should soften margarine and mix with peanut butter while the patient is breaking crackers into crumbs. Then the softened mixture and dry milk are mixed thoroughly in the bowl. Raisins, nuts and dates are added and mixed. The mixture is shaped into little balls by the patient and rolled in the cracker crumbs.

Fruit Compote

This is a simple dessert to prepare and you can vary the fruits to suit tastes. It is served with whipped cream which the patient can prepare. The caregiver should open the can of pineapples, put the fruit on a plate and save half of the liquid.

Seedless white grapes
A crisp apple
Pineapple chunks
2 mandarin oranges

The apple is peeled and diced and the mandarin oranges are separate into segments. Then the grapes, apple and mandarin orange pieces are mixed together with the pineapple juice. The fruit compote is chilled and served topped with whipped cream.

Crafts

Crafts

Craftwork is a creative activity and forms an integral part of many activity programs in hospital and day-care facilities for elderly people. With proper planning and safety measures, craftwork can also be a therapeutic and enjoyable activity for the patient at home. As with other activities, crafts should be chosen with the capabilities of the patient in mind.

- Crafts are suitable only for the person who can concentrate long enough to be able to follow the sequence of steps involved.

- The craft project must be carefully selected. Specifically, it should be simple enough so it will be completed by the patient rather than by the caregiver.

- Crafts which entail only a few large, easily manipulated components work best.

- It is important that the project be quick to complete. Otherwise, the patient will become restless because her attention span is limited.

- Only crafts which are adult in kind should be attempted since making fun figures or other childish objects will do little to raise the patient's self-esteem.

- Abstract projects should be avoided since they will be outside the patient's range of comprehension. The patient will be better able to relate to a structured project with well defined steps.

- It is helpful to have a ready-made model object which the patient can see and examine. This will help him visualize or imagine the end product. Introduce the steps involved one at a time. Keep in mind that even with a demonstration and ready-made model, there is no guarantee that a similar finished product will always materialize. It is in the **doing** that fulfillment occurs, rather than in the end product of a project.

Making Craftwork Hazard - Free

The patient will need continuous supervision during craftwork. He may lose the ability to discriminate between what is and what is not edible, so it is essential that all materials used be nontoxic. The caregiver must scrutinize projects thoroughly to check that all possible hazards are eliminated. For example, does the project involve the use of small objects such as coins, marbles or buttons? Is the patient prone to putting things in his mouth? If so, this information must be made available to all those involved in activities so that risk can be eliminated. Patients who are allowed to work with materials such as needles, scissors and glue must be able to use them appropriately and even then, they must have supervision.

Collage Ideas

Making a simple collage involves gathering magazines, selecting pictures, cutting them out, and arranging and pasting them on blank paper. This is a most suitable craft activity for the A.D. patient because it can be broken into separate, simple steps and requires little effort or skill. Collage-making is also a relatively clean and quiet activity which can be an individual or group project.

Treasure old magazines since they are full of collage material. Search through them for pictures that will help illustrate a particular theme. Gardening and cooking publications will provide a supply of colorful pictures. Under supervision the patient can cut these out and store them in a box specially for collage materials. To make the collage, the patient selects pictures of a certain theme and arranges them on a sheet of paper or cardboard.

Seasonal Collage This collage will help reinforce awareness of time and year. An Easter collage in the springtime colors of green, yellow, pink and lavender can be made quite easily just from pictures. Seasonal themes also provide good conversation material for the patient. Travel brochures, calendars and advertisements are ideal sources for summer, autumn or winter collage pictures.

Food Collage A collage of favorite foods can be made quite easily by pasting or taping colorful magazine pictures onto heavy cardboard.

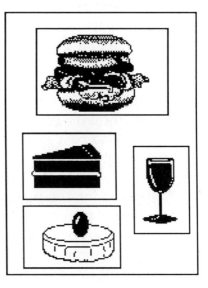

Events Collage The "event" themes are endless. Weddings, births, graduations, and moving house are some of the special events which may be significant to the patient. The event can be assembled from colorful pictures into collage form.

People Collage This collage could be of famous people, people working in different occupations, people involved in different sports, or playing different musical instruments. It might be a collage of people from different places. The possibilities are many and varied. A places collage is also a nice project. Be creative!

Scrapbooks

Scrapbooks centering on various themes may be made quite easily and will give many hours of enjoyment after completion. Magazines, newspapers, cards and photographs are good sources for pictures.

Family Scrapbook Mementos of family celebrations such as births and weddings, and pictures of places lived in can form the basis of a family scrapbook. This will also be a good memory prompter for the patient.

Hobby Scrapbook Special interest magazines can provide many colorful pictures for a scrapbook devoted to an old hobby or pastime. Themes may include sports, stamps, sailing, and gardening. It might even be favorite comic strips, or a newspaper recipe corner the patient collected.

Nature Scrapbook Pictures of birds, flowers, trees and animals may be cut from magazines, catalogs and Christmas cards. Actual objects may be used where appropriate; flowers, for example, can be collected, pressed and mounted in a scrapbook. Wildlife associations may be able to supply bird, animal, tree, and wildflower resource books for nature scrapbooks.

Season's Book A special book may be started at the beginning of the season. Here the patient can be helped to record dates of special outings, family activities, etc. Photographs may facilitate recall along with mementos like ticket stubs and programs.

Craft Ideas from Outings

The patient can record outings through simple craft work. As well as providing fun and therapy, these projects may also help the patient to remember the outing.

Mobiles A woodland mobile can be made from leaves, horsechestnuts, pine cones, pebbles, sticks and other small specimens collected on a journey out of doors. These simple nature materials can then be tied to a clothes hanger with different lengths of string, thread or yarn.

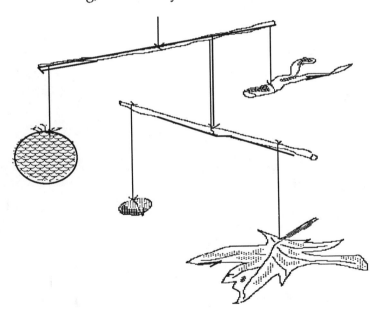

Alternatively, the woodland specimens could be stuck to wide masking tape and hung from any kind of rod.

Rubbings   Rubbing is similar to tracing except that the finished design is more shaded, and has a slightly three dimensional look. Here are a few things that take rubbings well: leaves, engraved signs, coins, the bark of a tree. Shelf paper, rice paper or onionskin typing paper can be laid over the object to be rubbed. The texture can be recorded on paper by rubbing back and forth over the textured surface with a pencil, crayon, or chalk.

The finished product may be displayed on a door, pasted into a scrapbook, or made part of a collage.

Gardening

Gardening

Gardening has long been thought of as a healing or therapeutic activity. In essence, it involves caring for a form of life and creating something of visual beauty. Since gardening stimulates memory through the use of all five senses— seeing, hearing, smelling, touching and sometimes tasting, it is well suited to the person with memory loss.

Select gardening activities which will require just enough attention for the patient to feel occupied, without becoming tired or feeling tied down. Everyday chores such as mowing the lawn, leaf raking and weeding can be done easily enough with some help and supervision. But keep in mind that if the work takes too long and becomes overwhelming, it loses its therapeutic value. Here are some ideas for simple and creative gardening projects.

Plant a Terrarium

When a clear plastic or glass container is filled with soil and plants and covered to form a miniature landscape, it is called a terrarium. Easy and inexpensive to make, the terrarium will add a pretty touch to the patient's room and give her something pleasant to look at. When friends visit it will make a fine conversation piece as it is such a novelty and tends to arouse curiosity. The terrarium when finished takes on the major responsibility for controlling its interior temperature and keeping the moisture level constant. The rest is up to you and the patient.

Plants   Decide on the plants you want to grow in the terrarium—you can plant a woodland, desert or flower-garden. Just keep in mind the full-grown plant size, how it grows, and where it likes to grow.

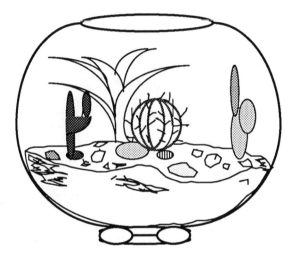

Container   Select a container, preferably one of clear plastic and as close to colorless as possible. The most common terrariums are planted in unused fish bowls, brandy snifters or apothecary jars. The more unusual the container, the more intriguing the terrarium will be.

Involve the patient in turning the terrarium about once a week and in watering it very occasionally.

Window Box Flowers

Flower boxes are very attractive and like terrariums, they are easy to care for. The patient may be able to help select the seeds and tend to the flower box once sown. Even the patient who is wheelchair-bound will be able to tend the window box flowers if they are within reach.

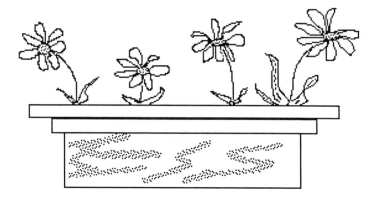

Decide on the flowers you want to grow. Your choice will depend on window exposure, room temperature and the space available. Start your flowers from seed or buy bedding plants. Once the plants are in place, put a layer of peat moss on top of the soil to keep it moist and cool.

Use a memory aid to remind the patient when plants need watering. A 3 x 5 index card with large, clearly typed instructions will be useful along with prompting from a family member.

Indoor Vegetable Garden

Try raising a plum or cherry tomato plant in a large flower pot—it works! Keep the plant in a sunny spot for as long as possible. Have the patient water it thoroughly every day. When the plant is about ten inches tall, stake it and keep it trained to the support while it grows.

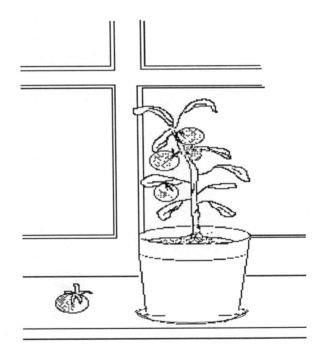

Indoor Herb Garden

You can grow lots of fresh herbs on a bright
kitchen windowsill all year round. As well as
looking nice, herbs smell good and will make
the room feel clean and bright. They will provide
a focus for the patient and stimulate the senses.
Like the terrarium, the herb garden is sure to
make a fine conversation piece. It does well with
very little care which the patient can give with
some supervision and prompting. A memory
card with instructions printed in large type
should be left by the herb garden.

Basil, dill and rosemary are three herbs that can
be easily grown from seeds or bedding plants.
Use separate clay pots for each individual herb
with its name clearly marked on it.

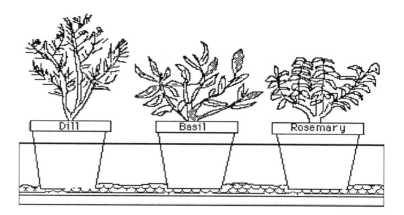

Put the pots into trays holding about an inch of
pebbles. Pour in just enough water to cover the
pebbles. Place the tray on a sunny windowsill.

Solo Activities

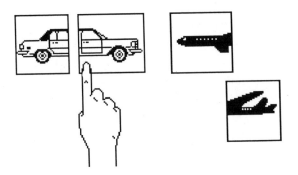

Solo Activities

Solo activities can be designed for the Alzheimer's patient so they demand little input from the caregiver. They are ideal to keep the patient occupied while the caregiver attends to other tasks. Like many other activities, they are so simple that they are often overlooked.

Reading

If the patient is still able to read, large-type books and magazines will be the most suitable. The subject matter should not be long or complex. Your local library is a good source for large-type publications. Popular magazines such as *Readers Digest, Sunshine Magazine* and *Guideposts* are available in large-type editions. Also of benefit are talking books and magazines, publications which are recorded on disc or tape. Many libraries have a wide selection available for circulation, including *Senior Citizen* and *Harvest Years*.

Large picture books are also very popular with Alzheimer's patients. Simple, uncluttered picture books work best and many hours of satisfaction can be derived from scanning the pictures of popular children's books. Collection books of famous comic strip characters can also provide quiet enjoyment.

Television

Some patients still enjoy watching TV even though they may have difficulty following the story-line. Others may find television threatening and so it is important to monitor viewing.

By observing how the patient responds to various programs, you will be able to chart what is suitable and stimulating for her. Action-packed programs are best avoided.

If used correctly, TV can become a useful resource and be of benefit to the patient. As well as its entertainment value, television has much potential for rekindeling old interests. A lifelong interest in classical music, for example, may be restimulated by viewing concerts or ballet. Someone who had an interest in athletics may have this interest revitalized by watching sports. The most popular programs tend to be :

- Comedy
- Children's educational programs
- Wildlife and sports

Winding
Winding a ball of yarn or a spool of thread is an activity well within the grasp of many patients. Unraveling old knitted garments is also an activity which many families find popular.

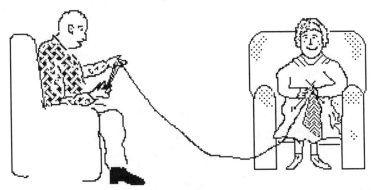

Shelling   One caregiver told of her relative getting long
periods of enjoyment from shelling nuts.
Friends brought bags of nuts to be shelled, so
the chore could be carried out to the benefit of
the A.D. patient and the visitor! In this activity,
provide a small bowl for the shelled nuts and
another for the shells.

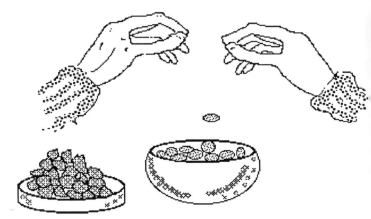

Sorting   Sorting buttons according to shape, size or color
and putting them into bags can be a useful
activity. Some patients may be able to sort
them according to material, with metal, plastic
and cloth ones being tipped into separate jars.
This activity must be carefully supervised.

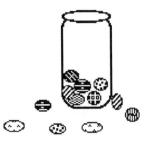

Coins (dimes, nickels, quarters and pennies) can be sorted and put into separate jars. This activity can keep the patient engrossed while at the same time offering a service to you.

There are endless ways in which old keys may be sorted: the thick ones separated from the slender; the long from the short.

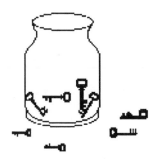

Playing cards may be sorted according to numbers, colors or suit. Postage stamps may be sorted for charity.

Encourage the patient to help you sort and match clothing before and after your weekly laundry. Perhaps he can help you separate white and dark colors, or maybe sort clothing according to fabrics. When the wash is done, the patient may be able to help out in sorting clothes of all different sizes and in matching and pairing socks. There are many other simple household chores that involve some element of sorting which the patient may be able to carry out.

Lacing   Simple lacing kits are available which can provide a quiet activity. One kit referred to in the appendix includes six ready-to-lace felt puppets, safety needles, yarn and colorful remnants to cut and lace.

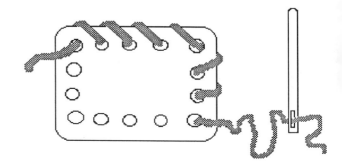

Stringing   Large colored wooden beads or blocks can be strung on a piece of yarn. A kit for this activity will include ready-to-string colored pieces and some yarn.

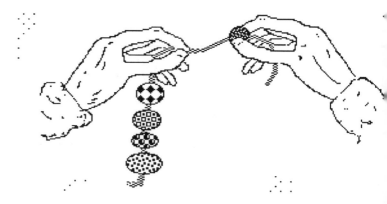

Solo Games

Many childrens educational games may be easily adapted to suit the Alzheimer's patient. As with all activities, they should be geared to the patients capabilities; simple games which have a few large components are the most suitable. Following are some ideas for solo games and similar versions of these are available from a number of toy manufacturers.

Matching   A series of cards are assembled to form a matching activity. Here, simple objects that relate to each other can be paired off, for example, a dog with a bone or a telephone with a receiver. Or, as in the examples below, two cards can be matched to form a single object.

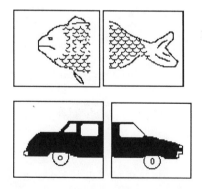

You can also make your own matching cards. Again, look to magazines for pictures and ideas.

**Sequence
Cards**   A series of cards can be arranged in sequence to
tell a story, each scene being made from 2 or 3
sequence cards. Themes for sequencing games
are numerous and the game has a short attention demand which makes it suitable for
Alzheimer's patients.

Pegboards   Working with pegboards helps to develop fine
motor control. There are many varieties of pegboards available. The most suitable pegs are
those which are large and easy-to-handle and
have a shoulder which gives a positive stop and
helps them fit snugly into the pegboard.

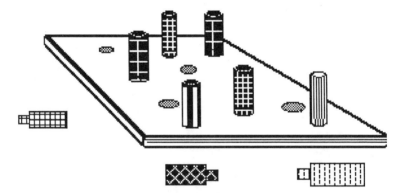

Family Games

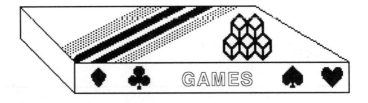

Family Games

When the family clan is together, make time for sharing through simple games. You may want to designate one evening a week as family night and have one or two relatives visit. Try to make family night the same each week so that family members will keep that night free when making individual plans.

Simple Games

There are many simple parlor games which the A.D. patient may be able to play. Games should be short and not demand much concentration.

Bingo   **Number Bingo.** A simplified version of Bingo with only the numbers 1 to 12 can be played to bring the game within the confused person's memory span. Here, each card has 4-6 numbers in large, easy-to-read print.

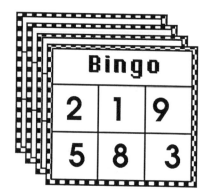

Picture Bingo. In picture bingo each person has a card with less than five easily identifiable pictures on it. The more personally relevant the pictures are, the better. The winner is the first to match all his pictures.

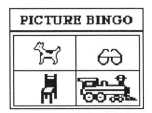

Money Bingo. Some patients may be able to play Money Bingo where coins are matched with their money values.

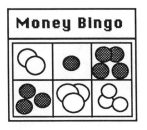

Charades   Word games can be played with letter cards, turning up say the letter E and asking the patient to name a word beginning with it. A game of charades can give practice in word-finding, body part identification and social interaction. For example, 'name a part of the body beginning with E.'

Shape Puzzles

These are games where a number of plastic or wooden shapes are fitted into corresponding holes in a board. They can spark off a discussion on shapes: squares, triangles, circles, e.g. " Show me another triangle. Point to the two circles." Colors can also be discussed, e.g. " Find another the same color as this—What else is green?" "Have you any clothes the same color as this?"

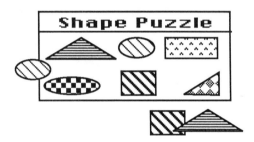

Jigsaws

Jigsaw puzzles can provide family members with a useful and fun activity. Puzzles with just a few large interlocking or magnetic pieces will be suitable for the patient with poor coordination. It is important that the jigsaw theme be adult in kind and within the patient's interest range. Keep a picture of the finished product in view and refer to it from time to time.

Lotto You can make lotto games quite easily using a large piece of paper or cardboard as your lotto board. Trace about six squares on the lotto board and stick on pictures. Mount similar pictures on stiff cardboard pieces for matching.

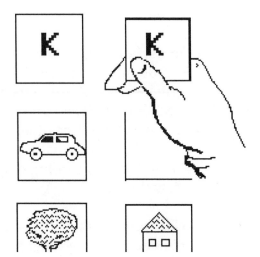

Activities Involving Children

With their spontaneity and uninhibited ways, young children are often a source of joy to the Alzheimer's patient. Children tend to have access to healing energies not available to the average adult. Programs such as **Project Joy** (joining older and younger) in Oakland utilize this by having children visit their day-care centers.

In the home, the playful presence of children can do much to lighten the atmosphere and bring a sense of fun to the patient's life. Children can take part in the activities above and in many of the other activities described in this book. You may want to prepare the child beforehand by reading one of the books suggested for children in Appendix A.

Children can share their interests with the patient. They can bring home a pet to visit or share a stamp collection, book or game. Perhaps they could share a tape-recording of a concert, church service, school program or band recital. Some children enjoy bringing treats such as candy or snacks to share. If there are older children in the family, they may be able to help the patient maintain ties with friends by reading cards and letters for her and helping her place phone calls.

Reminiscence

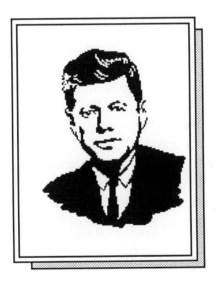

Reminiscence

Reviewing the past is a process that is believed to occur in all persons in the later years of their lives. Many elderly people have vivid memories of their past and can recall life events with remarkable clarity. People with profound memory loss often enjoy recounting their life stories to anyone who is willing to listen. Families may have difficulty in understanding how an Alzheimer's relative who cannot remember his own age or what he had for his last meal, can still recount a story from his childhood in detail. The reason has to do with the nature of memory loss in the disease. Loss of memory for recent events is usually profound, so that individuals may have difficulty remembering the previous sentence in a conversation, or the story line of a television movie. But long-term memory, that is memory of events in the distant past, may remain relatively intact, particularly throughout the early stages of the disease.

Group reminiscence sessions are now used in many nursing homes and day-care facilities which specialize in the care of victims of Alzheimer's disease. They provide participants with an opportunity to relive some of the past experiences of their lives. Families too can use reminiscence on a one-to-one basis with their memory-impaired relative at home.

Reminiscence has been found to be a successful
activity for victims of Alzheimer's disease for
a number of reasons:

- Reminiscence is a relatively non-threatening
  activity as it capitalizes on long-term
  memory, and patients usually feel secure in
  talking about the past.

- Exploring the past can serve as a substitute
  for active experience.

- Reminiscence can help to validate the
  contributions the patient has made
  throughout his life.

Activities Involving Reminiscence

Activities involving reminiscence call upon the
patient's skills or interests of long ago and in so
doing, help to validate his life contributions,
interests and feelings. The focus on validation is
central to reminiscence. It helps acknowledge
the person the patient was, and continues to be,
despite the disease process.

Focusing on the past is a central part of reminiscence. In many of the activities outlined here, use
is made of old items, books, pictures, records —
aids to provoke memories and recall experiences. Articles which have lain in basements for
years, unused and unnoticed, take on a new
importance as they are used for reminiscence.

Make a Life Collage

Involve the patient in making his own life collage. It can include a written biographical sketch mentioning his former occupation, achievements and interests. Photos of family and friends and pictures of places lived in can be included. Post the collage in an obvious part of the patient's room. It will provide a good topic of conversation for visitors who are often unsure of what to talk about.

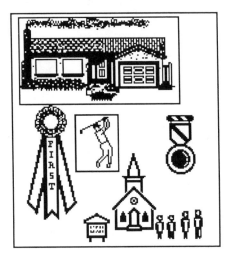

Materials Needed:

- Large sheet of mounting board
- Cellophane Tape
- Safety Scissors
- Written biographical sketch /family tree
- Photographs

Make a Memory Book

A memory book can provide a written and pictorial record of the patient's life. It can be compiled with the help of the patient and at a pace conducive to reminiscing.

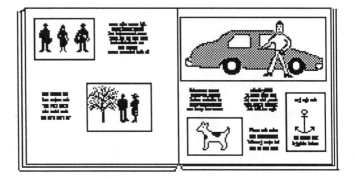

Family members at all levels can become involved, working with the patient and slowly piecing together the highlights of his life. Pictures, headlines and news items from old newspapers and magazines can be pasted in where appropriate, to put the patient's life in context.

The local library or historical society may have additional material which would help to illustrate what was happening locally during the patient's life. If there are children in the family, leafing through the memory book with the patient will help them to share something from his past. On completion, the memory book will provide the patient with hours of passive entertainment.

Materials needed for memory book :

- Large spiral notebook or scrapbook
- Marker pens or crayons
- Cellophane Tape
- Old newspapers
- Magazines and cataloges
- Postcards

- Written accounts of experiences, events and achievements
- Written accounts by family members of special memories they have of the patient

- Photographs of house of birth, parents, grandparents, cousins, siblings etc.
- Photographs of memorable moments: graduation, wedding, birth of children, retirement etc.

Make a Memory Box

Help the patient to make a memory box consisting of objects from his past. Hunt for early "junk" in attics, basements and store-rooms. Any memorabilia from the patient's life will probably be useful—trophies, autograph books, postcards, stamp albums, report cards, school books, even diaries and letters belonging to the patient. The memory box can include very old items from the patient's childhood.

Placed beside the patient's chair, the memory box will provide a stimulus for discussion.

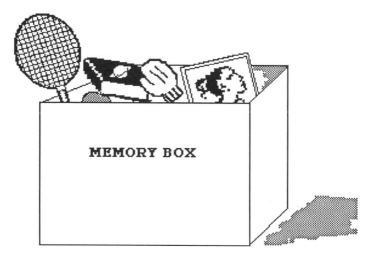

Family members can pay attention to what stimulates his curiosity most to get clues for further themes for conversation. By exploring the memory box with their relative, children can learn more about "the old days."

The memory box provides a wonderful focus for conversation for visitors who can draw on it to talk about the past. Friends may even be able to add old photographs and various knick-knacks when they visit. For the patient who is conscious of his memory loss, the memory box makes visits from friends easier by providing a conversation piece.

Make a Photo Album

Old photographs are a wonderful resource for reminiscence and browsing through a photo album will provide an enjoyable activity for patient and caregiver.

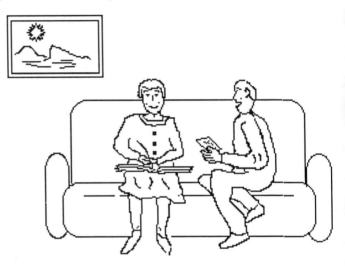

The patient's history or that of the family can be pieced together pictorially using family photo albums. Families often label photos to help the patient remember relatives and close friends. Learn which photos are most important to the patient so he can carry them around in a pocket if he wishes. As conversation pieces, photos are excellent.

Home Movies and Slides

Old home movies, taken when family members were younger, provide an excellent stimulus for reminiscence and "then" and "now" comparisons. Likewise, slides of places and people once familiar to the patient can evoke memories of very distant times. Families which have these visual materials should recognize their usefulness in eliciting memories.

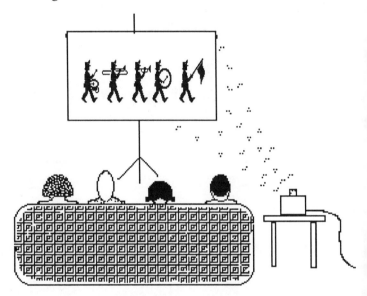

VCR equipment gives an opportunity for viewing films at opportune times without commercial interruptions and videos of favorite old-time movies could be hired occasionally. A special family night for viewing movies and slides can be arranged every so often.

Books   "Then" and "Now" books are invaluable for discussing how things have changed during the patient's lifetime. Many towns and cities have pictorial books showing local places and familiar landmarks as they were over the years.

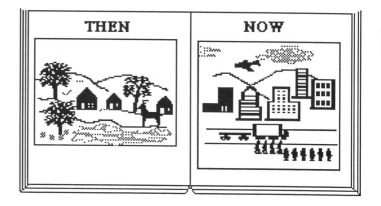

Where a book of this kind isn't available, the family very easily can put their own together. Copies of "Then" and "Now" photos are often available from libraries. Look for pictures which might have some relevance for the patient— an old cinema, town hall, park, farmer's market, favorite street. These can be compiled to make either a book or a collage and will provide the stimulus for reminiscence. Children will enjoy taking part in this activity.

Personality Parade Make a scrapbook (or a series of them) with pictures and photographs of people who were famous in the patient's younger days. You might begin with movie stars. As prompts, titles of particular films, songs or catch-phrases can be written in to accompany photographs. Reminiscing over these pictures, perhaps with a child, can provide the patient with hours of passive entertainment. You can also look for pictures of famous people in:

- Sports
- Politics
- Movies
- Music
- Military

Place the Picture Compile a scrapbook of pictures of "then" and "now" objects with the patient. The following antique objects contrasted with pictures of their more modern-day equivalents will provoke memories, laughter and plenty discussion !

Steam engine	Old iron
Washboard	Bathtub
Oil lamp	Lantern
Old bicycle	Old juke box
Kitchen jug	Dresser
Cable car	Old telephone
Old radio	Old motorbike
Pocket watch	Gas lamp

Musical Memories

The patient can be entertained for hours by listening to music on a portable player with headphones, while allowing family members some respite and a chance to get on with daily chores. Particular songs may be selected to stimulate memories of various stages of the life cycle. Listening to these songs can help the patient to get in touch with parts of his past and help him come more alive in the present.

Listening to old love songs is popular. People can hear their own experiences through love songs; often they are a validation of one's own triumphs and sadnesses in the court of love. Many people have a favorite love song which lasts throughout life. It may be reminiscent of a particular phase in a relationship; special moments associated with the song will help to recreate memories. Old classics may be located with the help of a local record store or library.

Here are a few ideas:

Let Me Call You Sweetheart
When I Grow Too Old To Dream
Somewhere My Love
Give Me A Little Kiss (Will You?)
Be My Love
Are You Lonesome Tonight
I Love You Truly
Heart Of My Heart
Release Me
Goodnight Sweetheart

Outings   An occasional outing will keep the patient from feeling isolated and help him stay oriented to the world around him. Visits should be made to places once familiar to the patient, maybe the street where he worked, a favorite ball park or beach. You can help the patient by pointing out new developments en route. Streets and buildings being remodelled or torn down provide great cues for reminiscence.

It is most important that outings be non threatening for the patient. Places visited should be stress-free and quiet.

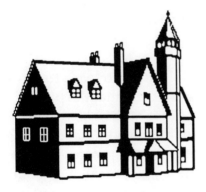
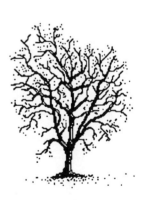

Reminiscence Discussions

Reminiscing feels safe for people with Alzheimer's disease because they are more in control when talking about the past. Remember though, that reminiscing with your relative is <u>not</u> the same as encouraging him to live in the past. The following guidelines are worth remembering as you reminisce with the patient.

- Help keep facts accurate by relating them to the past as opposed to the present.

- Discuss topics in a quiet, unhurried way, giving the patient ample time to respond.

- Use clear enunciation and a good deal of expression. Give cues and prompts where necessary

- Use a tangible focus for each topic—something concrete that the patient can see such as a photograph or souvenir. This will help to prompt memories and will remind the patient of what the conversation is about. If, for example, you're talking about vacations, have a selection of relevant pictures available from travel brochures. Using the family photo album will enhance a discussion about relatives.

- Be sensitive to difficult issues and emotions which may arise.

Themes for Reminiscence

Build a bank of themes for reminiscence. From the following suggestions, select those which the patient can relate to best.

Home   Where was your first home? Did you move often? Why? What was your favorite house?

School   Where did you attend your first school? What was the school like? Who taught you? Who was your favorite teacher? What was your favorite subject?

Pets   Did you ever have a pet? What did you call it? How did you decide on its name? Would you like to have a pet now? (Show pictures of pets which people have: hamsters, cats, dogs, birds, fish, turtles.)

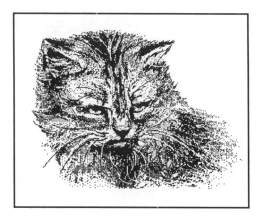

Names Do you recall the names of childhood friends? Who gave you your name— your mother or father? Is there a special name you would like to have been called by? What is your favorite name? What names don't you like? Why?

Pastimes What was your favorite pastime ? Did you ever go fishing? Sailing ? Who went with you ? Where did you go ?

Sports Did you have a favorite sport? What teams did you follow? Who were the stars?

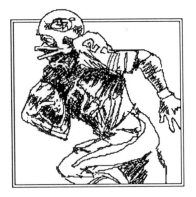

Happy Days Do you recall a day that was happier than all others? Describe it. What kinds of things make you happy now?

Halloween How did you celebrate Halloween when you were a child? Was it a special holiday for you? What was your favorite Halloween game? Did you ever go to a fancy-dress Halloween ball?

Vacations   Where you went — who you went with. Interesting sights, special moments, funny incidents. Souvenirs, gifts you brought back. What kind of holiday would you like to have gone on. Your best vacation. (Use pictures, photos, posters and brochures.)

Books   Favorite books: mysteries, adventure stories, animal stories, how-to-books, cookbooks, picture books. What books do you like to look at now? Did you read Mark Twain when you were young.

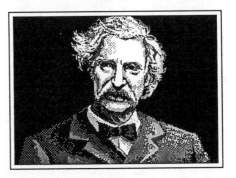

Food   Do you have a favorite food? What kind of food did you eat during the war?

Television   Tell me about your first TV. What were your favorite programs? Can you name the personalities? What was it like without TV?

Transport   What special transport did you use growing up?
Did you drive, own a car, have a bike? What
kind was your first car? Pictures of various
modes of transportation will aid discussions.

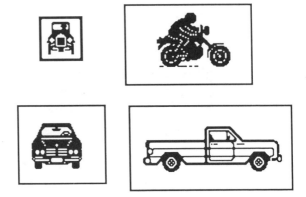

Romance   Your first romance. Your first dance, date. How
and where you met your wife. Activities and
places you enjoyed while dating. When did you
fall in love? What qualities attracted you to one
another? How long did your engagement last?
Any stories about your courtship? How you
proposed? Tell me about your wedding. Where
did you go on your honeymoon?

Children   At what age did you have your first child? How
you decided on the name.

Gifts   Were you ever given a gift that you have always
treasured? Why was it special? Describe some
gifts you have given.

Work   What you worked at. Tell about your first paycheck. Who worked with you? What did family members work at?

Prices   Discuss how prices and incomes have changed over the years. Cost of basic commodities—tea, sugar, pint of milk, bread, butter, meat. Price of a stamp, local phonecall, children's toys. Price of a glass of beer, clothes, travel. How expensive was it to go to a movie, to dine out, to rent an apartment? How much did it cost to have a haircut, buy a plot of land, a house?

The Depression   What age were you when it struck? What were you working at then? How did it affect you and your family? The community? What are some of the memories you have of that period?

Fashions   Were you fashion-conscious? What type of clothes did you like to wear? Did you have a choice or did you wear hand-me-downs? Show pictures of changing fashions down through the years, from bell-bottoms to mini-skirts. These can produce fascinating reminiscences.

Appendix A

Suggested Reading for Caregivers

Mace, N. & Rabin, P. THE 36-HOUR DAY.
New York: Warner Books, 1981.
This is an excellent readable explanation of
many problem behaviors and symptoms in
Alzheimer's disease. Highlighted are the emo-
tional implications for the spouse and adult
child, as well as the importance of supportive
help from relatives, friends, self-help groups,
and professional groups. Also dealt with are
legal, financial and placement issues that every
family must face. Essentially directed at the
family, the book is also a useful guide for
professionals.

Gwyther, Lisa P. (1985) **Care of Alzheimer's
Patients: A Manual for Nursing Home Staff**
This book offers practical assistance to both
professionals and family caregivers on managing
Alzheimer's patients with behavioral problems.
The author shares vignettes on particular behaviors and suggests ways to cope and to strengthen
effective care techniques. Though written for
nursing home staff, the book is readily adaptable
to adult day care programs. Available for $6.95
from any local chapter of ADRDA.

Kushner, Harold S. **When Bad Things Happen
to Good People**
New York: Shocken Books, 1981.

Suggested Reading for Children

Young, Alida, E. **What's wrong with daddy?**
Ohio: Willowisp Press 1986.
This is a fiction piece for a popular audience
which attempts to capture the feelings of an
adolescent whose parent is afflicted with AD.

Guthrie, Donna. **Grandpa doesn't know it's me.**
Published by Human Sciences Press & ADRDA
This book describes a family's experiences of
coping with Alzheimer's disease and is useful in
helping young children deal with the conflicting
emotions serious family illness may generate.
The book is available through ADRDA's chapters, the ADRDA national office, and bookstores.

Noyes, Lin E. **What's wrong with my grandma?**
Published by ADRDA & Northern Virginia
Chapter.
Available from 2OO East Broad St. #I,
Falls Church, Virginia 22O46. (7O3) 534-8466.

Appendix B

Activity Resources

The following children's educational games may be adapted for use with the Alzheimer's patient. They are available from :

Warren's Educational Supplies,
Main Office,
980 W. San Bernadino Rd.
Covina,
Ca. 91722

Stringing
Big beads for stringing and sorting. Big, bright wooden beads in 7 shapes and colors can be strung to form countless patterns and designs. Includes 30 nontoxic beads and string. The largest bead is 2" long.
ET-4105 $9.95

Sewing
Sew-a-Foam: Simple step-by-step kit includes all the materials for sewing pictures from patterns. Four 10" blocks,12 pattern cards 9"x 9"; yarn in 8 colors , 4 safety needles.
ID 6094 $17.95

Sewing Cards.This set of 32 sewing design cards includes 4 safety needles and enough colored yarn to create 16 different preprinted designs of familiar objects.
ID 6095 $7.I5.

Lacing   Lacing Shapes.
A delightful primary lacing activity. Nine shiny
shapes of colorful, heavy chipboard (4 to 5"
long) with nine non-kink laces in various colors.
No needles required.
LR 2561 $5.50

Lace a pet puppet.
Ready-to-lace felt puppets. Kit includes three
animal shapes, three plastic safety needles, yarn
and plenty of colorful shapes and remnants to
cut and glue.
LR 2511 $6.25

Sequencing   These storyboards consist of panels and an inlay
Sets   frame; the objective is to arrange sequences and
describe activities. Each 12" scene is made from
2, 3 or 4 sequence cards.
Complete package (72) sets $19.95
Group I - Community Helpers $ 6.95
Group II - Growing Things $ 6.95
Group III - Machines & more $ 6.95

Matching   Object Match. 10 self-correcting wood plaques
match 2 objects that relate to each other such as
a dog with a bone, a telephone with a receiver
etc. The objects are simple and silk-screened.
Each plaque is 5" x3".
No. MTC 249 $6.75.

Things That Go Together.
This set was designed to stimulate discussion of matching objects.
Set I contains 30cards, $5.95. Set 2 contains 16 more familiar pairs, $5.95.

Feel & Match Textures.
Twelve 3 1/2" disks of six different texture materials, such as felt, plastic, rubber, chipboard, etc. Can be used for sensory stimulation exercise.
LR 2206. $4.25

Dominoes

Beginner Sets. Twelve piece beautifully crafted woodblock dominoe sets to sort, match and classify.

Geometric shapes	JI 4001
Animals	JI 4003
Foods	JI 4004
	$5.95 each

Shape & Size dominoes
The 24 pieces in this set are printed in two colors on durable plastic and offer a visual perception activity requiring players to match shape and size combinations.
T 528   Set $8.85.

Lotto   Color Lotto
11" square inlay wood tray with three sets of 9 colored squares for developing color recognition.   J700005 $8.95.

Learning by doing Lotto Games.
Players exercise object identification, language, motor and special skills as they identify and match 16 lotto cards with the familiar objects on the18" x 18" plastic-coated game-board. Each lotto game may be played as a group game or as an individual activity. Games on various themes. $7.50 each

Pegboard   Easy Grip Pegs
Contoured for rigid hands and for special education, these pegs help develop fine motor control. The shoulder on each peg insures a positive stop when inserted into a pegboard. Pegs come in six colors and are designed for Jumbo Tactilmat Pegboards.
ID 6236 25 Pegs $6.25

Jumbo Holdtight Peg Sets.
These oversize colorful plastic pegs in five colors are perfect for rigid fingers. A 'shoulder' on the pegs gives a positive stop and helps them fit snugly into the pliable, indestructible rubber pegboards. The large pegboard is 17" square and has 100 holes. The small pegboard is 8" square with 25 holes.
No. MTC-875   100 Hole Pegboard $11.50
No. MTC-762   100 Hold-Tight Pegs $18.95

Inlay Puzzles All beginner inlay puzzles are available with coordination-building knobs which make it easier to manipulate pieces. Themes include Fruits, Vegetables and Table Setting, $7.95 each.

Bingo Color bingo: an appealing color recognition game that includes red, orange, yellow, brown, green, blue, pink and purple colors. $6.95

Money bingo: a stimulating, active way to play bingo. players simply match coins with money values. Features pennies, nickels and dimes in values from 3 cents to 50 cents. $6.95.

Number Bingo: Number Bingo features numerals 1-20 in large, easy-to-read print. $4.49.

The following games are available from **Eldergames,** a nonprofit company that specializes in developing, manufacturing and distributing games for people suffering from Alzheimer's Disease or other disorders that cause memory loss.

Feel 'n Fold is based on the worry bead concept. Soft colored fabrics of several interesting textures permit repetitive folding action that is a common characteristic of Alzheimer's patients. Recommended for agitated individuals as a soothing and stroking diversion.
Price $6.

Memory Joggers is a line of decks of oversized, easy-to-see, illustrated flash cards designed to stimulate recall. Illustrations are pegged to thematic categories, e.g., transportation, sports, tools of the trade. Each deck includes 25 cards. Price: $10 per deck.

Elder Trivia includes more than 250 memory teasing questions based on nostalgic events and organized into eight categories to amuse and stimulate: Famous people, Songs, Colors, Geographic Locations, Literature, Science, Entertainment and History. price $9.
For more information, write to:
> **Eldergames,**
> 11710 Hunters Lane,
> Rockville,
> MD 20852.

Music There are many collections of old-time favorite songs now available. Two excellent cassette tapes entitled **"Sing-A-Long Down Memory Lane"** include over 40 of the all-time favorites, along with a complete set of words. They are available at a cost of $10 and 50 cents handling charge from:
> **K & D Productions,**
> P.0. Box 803,
> Evansville,
> IN. 47708.

Appendix C
Organizations

The following organizations provide family members and caregivers with information about Alzheimer's disease, various care options and services. Contact the National ADRDA and get on their newsletter mailing list. They may also be able to put you in contact with a local chapter and support group.

National ADRDA
70 E. Lake Street,
Chicago,
Illinois 6060I.
(312) 853-3060
(800) 621-0379

Family Survival Project
1736 Divisadero Street,
San Francisco,
CA 94115.

Index

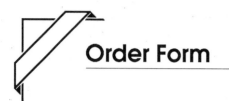

Order Form

Cottage Books,
2419 13th Avenue,
Oakland,
CA. 94606.

Please send me _____ copies of **" Failure-Free Activities for the Alzheimer's Patient"** @ $9.95 each.

Name: _____

Address:_____

City:_____ Zip: _____

Shipping and handling: $1.25 for first book , additional books 50¢ each.

Californians: Please add 65¢ sales tax.

Total Amount Enclosed : _____